GREGORY PAYAN AND
CASEY GALLAGHER

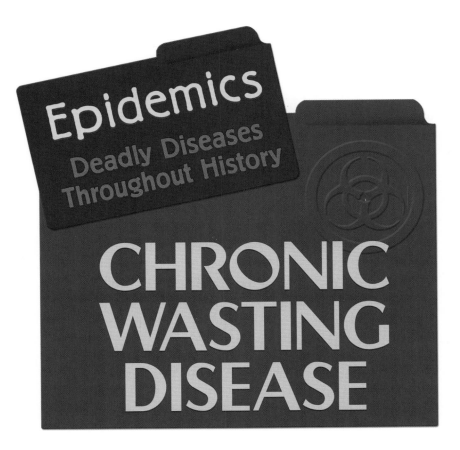

Epidemics
Deadly Diseases
Throughout History

CHRONIC
WASTING
DISEASE

The Rosen Publishing Group, Inc.
New York

Published in 2004 by The Rosen Publishing Group, Inc.
29 East 21st Street, New York, NY 10010

Library of Congress Cataloging-in-Publication Data

Payan, Gregory.
Chronic wasting disease / by Gregory Payan and Casey Gallagher.— 1st ed.
      p. cm. — (Epidemics: deadly diseases throughout history)
Summary: Describes CWD, a deadly disease that affects deer and elk, detailing its cause and symptoms, as well as research that is being done to control the epidemic and find a cure.
Includes bibliographical references and index.
ISBN 0-8239-4198-1 (lib. bdg.)
1. Chronic wasting disease—Juvenile literature. [1. Chronic wasting disease. 2. Diseases.] I. Gallagher, Casey. II. Title. III. Epidemics.
SF997.5.C46 P38 2003
573.8'639—dc21

                                                        2003001769

Manufactured in the United States of America

Cover image: A microscopic image of tissue damaged by chronic wasting disease

CONTENTS

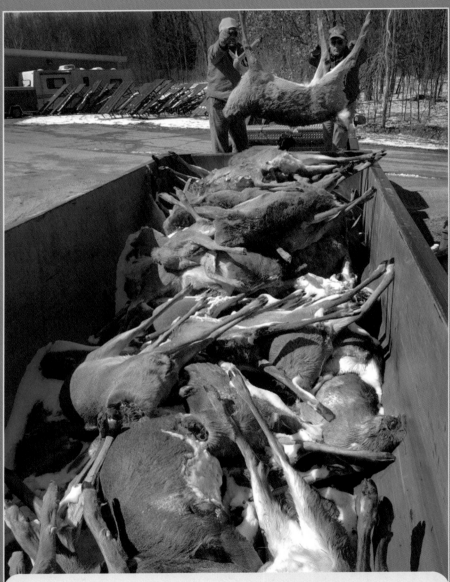

Chronic wasting disease is an illness that affects wildlife, including the deer pictured here that were ravaged during an outbreak in 2002.

INTRODUCTION

In 1967, deer in captivity began to die mysteriously in northeastern Colorado. A research facility was doing studies on captive mule deer. The facility had been conducting many experiments on local wildlife, including white-tailed deer, elk, sheep, and goats. In this particular study, Colorado State University graduate student Gene Schoonveld had begun a three-year project to determine why mule deer didn't digest hay and alfalfa during harsh winters in Colorado. In addition to the test animals that were bred for research, the Colorado Division of Wildlife provided him with four dozen deer from the wild to be kept in a separate 40-by-45-foot area. Soon after the study began, the deer began to mysteriously get sick and die.

Over the course of the study, approximately thirty-six deer died. All of the deer had similar symptoms. They would lose weight despite eating regularly and completely "waste away" before dying. This is the reason that later on, after the disease was identified, it was given the name chronic wasting disease. When examinations were performed on the dead deer, it was determined that they died from an inflammation of the intestinal tract. No one considered that the deer were dying from a mysterious disease that scientists had never seen before.

Since the deer were being studied and monitored, scientists were able to see strange behavior in the sick deer. The scientists found it odd that the deer were dying without an apparent reason, but they only thought that something was missing from the deer's diets. The scientists presumed that there was some-thing the deer got from their diets in the wild that they weren't getting in captivity. It was easy for them to say that the deer's diet was causing the problem, but maybe they missed other signs that something more serious was happening. The deer were drooling and grinding their teeth. They were also drinking very large amounts of water and urinating excessively.

Although their diet was suspected of making them sick, the deer were dying quickly after the onset of symptoms. If there was a dietary problem, wouldn't they be dying slowly as their bodies tried to make up for missing nutrients? Something else was occurring that was much more deadly. There were questions about the mysterious deaths, but not enough for scientists to conduct more tests, which they likely should have. Many years later, this would prove to be a terrible mistake.

THE BEGINNING

It is difficult to determine the exact beginnings of chronic wasting disease, or CWD. After all, as with most diseases, it's nearly impossible to determine when a disease began infecting people or animals. In most cases, scientists can only make their best guesses based on the information available. Although research can show when the disease was first identified, nobody can say for certain when CWD began to infect deer and elk.

Chronic Wasting Disease Affects the Brain

After the 1967 study, there were some questions left unanswered. But nobody could have

8

imagined the consequences of not conducting more tests on the sick deer. A series of events over the next few years would show how big a mistake the scientists had made.

In 1977, years after Gene Schoonveld's original study, Beth Williams, a young graduate student in Colorado, decided to look at the brain tissue from a deer that had died with the same symptoms as the deer in Dr. Schoonveld's study. An illness of the brain was not suspected years before, and therefore the brains of the sick animals were never examined. When Williams looked through the microscope, she saw that the brain tissue had tiny holes in it. It looked just like the brain of a sheep that had died from scrapie. Scrapie had been identified more than 200 years earlier as a disease that affects only sheep. Scrapie got its name from the strange behavior of the infected sheep. Sheep with scrapie will scrape their skin against hard objects until raw, as if trying to scratch an uncontrollable itch. Eventually, the sheep die.

Scrapie is a deadly disease that is classified as transmissible spongiform encephalopathy, or TSE. The word "spongiform" describes the spongelike condition of the brain when an animal or a person contracts a TSE. When someone or something is infected by a TSE, tiny holes form in the brain tissue. These holes are visible only through examination using a microscope. TSEs attack the brain and central nervous system, destroying healthy tissue. The victim loses physical and mental abilities as the disease progresses. Eventually, the victim dies.

CWD Is a TSE

After Beth Williams discovered that the brain tissue of the deer and the sheep were similar, she searched for another scientist to confirm her findings. She asked her mentor, Dr. Stuart Young, to look at the slide. Dr. Young agreed that the deer specimen looked like the specimen of a victim with a TSE. He, too, asked another expert to examine their findings, and a leading veterinarian confirmed their suspicions. CWD was not a disease that affected the intestines—it affected the brain. A major breakthrough in research had been made, but now that they knew it was a TSE, experts were more fearful than they were before. TSEs are always fatal, and very little is known about them.

Other TSEs

The three most widely known TSEs that can affect animals are scrapie, which has been identified in sheep for more than 200 years; bovine spongiform

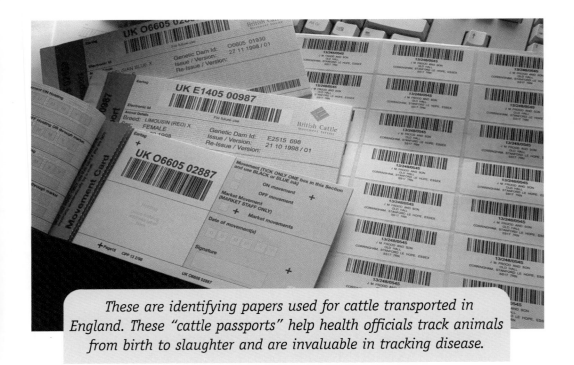

These are identifying papers used for cattle transported in England. These "cattle passports" help health officials track animals from birth to slaughter and are invaluable in tracking disease.

encephalopathy (BSE), otherwise known as mad cow disease; and CWD, which affects deer and elk. TSEs also can affect cats, mink, and some rodents. Two known TSEs can affect humans: Creutzfeldt-Jakob disease (CJD), which occurs naturally in about one out of every one million people, and variant CJD (vCJD), which has been linked to the mad cow disease outbreak in England. A victim gets vCJD by eating beef or beef products from a cow that had BSE. During the mad cow outbreak in England in the 1980s and 1990s, it is estimated that the British consumed nearly 750,000 infected cattle during a ten-year period. Although the British government insisted for years that no harm could occur from eating contaminated meat, they were wrong. To date, more than 100 people have died of vCJD.

How Did the Original Deer Get Sick?

So how did CWD begin to affect deer? At the Colorado research facility, a number of sheep and deer were held together in one big pen from 1968 to 1971. One theory is that over these years the agent that causes scrapie "jumped" from the infected sheep to the deer, possibly through shared food or the exchange of saliva. Experts think that this disease then grew into CWD in the research deer. Over the course of the study, the research deer would occasionally make contact with wild deer and elk that approached the pen. Since scientists believe the disease is spread through saliva and nose-to-nose contact, many feel this is one of the ways CWD was spread into the wild.

In a *Rocky Mountain News* article in 2002, Dr. Schoonveld said, "They [the deer] were in close proximity of the sheep for long periods of time and it was among those animals that the symptoms of CWD first showed up. My best guess as a biologist is those sheep had scrapie and in close confinement, something they wouldn't do in the wild—it jumped to the deer and infected them. I'm guessing it was prolonged nose-to-nose exposure between infected sheep and deer that may have led to the jump."

Many deer in captivity died of CWD during various studies throughout the 1970s. No one knew that the deer that died of CWD had a disease that was contagious to other healthy animals. At this time, scientists still thought the disease was related to the diet of the research deer. Many of the captive deer and their offspring that showed no signs of the mysterious disease were released back into the wild, just like the deer in Dr. Schoonveld's original study. Only years later would scientists learn that deer can have the

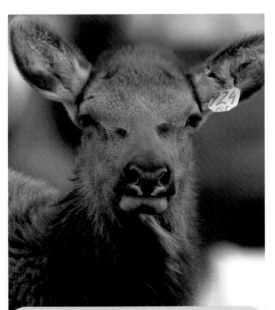

This elk in Colorado was tagged to identify it as a carrier of chronic wasting disease. The elk was put to sleep shortly after.

disease for years without showing symptoms. People involved in these studies unknowingly had risked infecting wild herds of deer by releasing research deer that may have been sick back into the wild.

1967
CWD is first recognized as a disease in mule deer at a research facility in Fort Collins, Colorado.

1977
Elizabeth Williams identifies CWD as a TSE, or transmissible spongiform encephalopathy.

1981
CWD is diagnosed in an elk that has died in the wild in Colorado.

1981
CWD is diagnosed in free-range deer in northeast Colorado.

1981
Surveillance for CWD in Colorado and Wyoming is started.

1982
Stanley Prusiner, microbiologist and neurologist, reports evidence that TSEs are caused by a self-replicating protein (prion).

1985
CWD is found in free-range deer and elk in southeastern Wyoming.

1996
The first case of CWD is discovered in a game farm in Saskatchewan, Canada. The elk had been imported from the United States.

2001
CWD is diagnosed in free-range deer in Nebraska and Saskatchewan.

2002
CWD is diagnosed in free-range deer in Wisconsin, New Mexico, South Dakota, and Illinois.

2001
CWD is diagnosed in a domestic elk herd in Kansas.

2002
CWD is diagnosed in a domestic deer herd in Alberta, Canada, and in a domestic elk herd in Minnesota.

1997–1999
CWD is diagnosed in domestic elk herds in South Dakota, Nebraska, Oklahoma, Colorado, and Montana.

2001
CWD is diagnosed in an elk imported from Canada to Korea in 1997.

2003
CWD is diagnosed in free-range deer in Utah.

2001
The United States Department of Agriculture (USDA) declares an animal emergency because of CWD in game farm elk.

CWD Is Found in the Wild

In 1981, a huge, beautiful bull elk was found dead of CWD in Colorado. It was the first known case of CWD outside of the research pens. CWD had gotten out and, most likely, could no longer be controlled. Not only were deer in the wild at risk, but it was now confirmed that elk were at risk as well. Nobody knew how far it had already spread or how much it would continue to.

Did scrapie jump the species barrier and become CWD in deer? Beth Williams, currently a professor of veterinary sciences at the University of Wyoming, explained in a 2002 article in the *Rocky Mountain News*, "While it's reasonable to assume such a jump occurred from sheep to deer, there is absolutely nothing to prove it. It's equally as plausible that CWD is a naturally occurring disease as well."

CWD could have been a naturally occurring disease in the wild for years. It could be that an animal or animals that were brought into the pen at CSU could have already had the disease and spread it among the other deer in the pen. Unlike in the wild, scientists could follow the disease as symptoms progressed in the research studies. We just don't know and likely never will.

2

CWD SPREADS LIKE WILDFIRE

From 1969 to 1996, the only confirmed cases of chronic wasting disease occurred in Wyoming and Colorado. Many people felt that since there were so few diagnosed cases, there was little to worry about. Now, all of a sudden, there is a lot more to fear. Since 1996, cases of CWD have been confirmed in Montana, Oklahoma, Kansas, Nebraska, Wisconsin, South Dakota, New Mexico, Illinois, Utah, and Canada. Recently in Minnesota, an infected elk was found in captivity. This worried scientists greatly because of the large number of white-tailed deer that live in Minnesota and the possibility that the infected elk could have had contact with deer. It has been suggested that the disease spreads most easily among white-tailed deer.

CWD Spreads Over Geographical Boundaries

National attention was given to the disease when it was discovered west of the Rockies and, subsequently, east of the Mississippi River in Wisconsin. How could infected animals have crossed the rugged Rocky Mountains or the Mississippi River? That this happened within the last few years is truly frightening to experts and government officials. After so many years of being isolated in Colorado and Wyoming, why is the disease being found far and wide, crossing geographical hurdles experts thought impossible?

Many people view elk ranching as the primary reason CWD has spread so far so quickly, and elk ranchers are often blamed for making the spread of CWD a crisis situation. How is this so? When kept on an elk ranch, elk are unnaturally bunched together. Anytime animals (or humans) are confined to a small area, it makes it easier for all contagious diseases to spread. Since many experts believe that CWD is spread through contact between animals, often through their saliva, it is reasonable to believe that when elk come to feed at man-made stations (as they do on elk farms), sick elk are infecting healthy elk. Contact with urine and feces is also believed to be a possible way to spread the disease, and ranching promotes such contact as well.

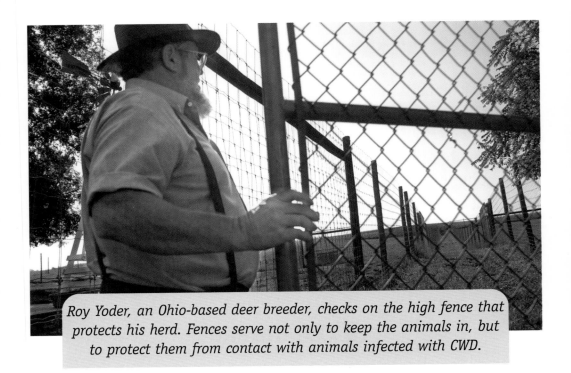

Roy Yoder, an Ohio-based deer breeder, checks on the high fence that protects his herd. Fences serve not only to keep the animals in, but to protect them from contact with animals infected with CWD.

Fences Provide Little Help

On ranches, elk are usually kept behind large wire fences. Deer and other animals can get over or under these fences and have contact with sick animals. Winds knock fences over, floods create openings underneath the fences, and snow piles up, allowing animals to climb over the fences. Wild animals can go in, and sick animals can go out into the wild, thus spreading the disease. While many have suggested double fences would help the problem, right now, very few ranches have them. Double fencing is expensive, and no one can agree on who should pay for it.

Most experts believe a second fence (about eight feet tall) outside the original perimeter, with wire in between posts, would help. They say the second fence would further prevent the disease from coming in or going out. Nobody is sure if the disease is being transmitted through fences, but in the end, it appears that the public's tax dollars will be paying for double fencing, which many hope will help stop the spread of disease.

Shipping of Elk Also Contributes to the Spread

Another factor that aids the spread of CWD is that captive elk are often shipped hundreds of miles as elk ranchers trade, purchase, and sell the animals to each other. Ranchers seek trophy bulls and try to maintain diversity in the herd. All these factors contribute to the spread of the disease. As the disease was rapidly spreading during the last few years, no laws existed to prevent animals from CWD herds from being transferred from state to state. Now, many state governments are enacting laws to block the movement of any captive deer or elk into state lands.

According to a 2002 article in the *Denver Post*, Dr. Bruce Cheesebro, leading researcher at the National Institutes of Health's Rocky Mountain laboratories, recently said, "People ask how this disease is spreading, and I say, 'by truck.' It is being moved around in these game farms and is leaking out into the wildlife. Until you close down the game farms, you can kill all the wildlife you want and you will not halt the spread of this disease."

Are Elk Farms Worth It?

Taxpayer money supplements these elk farms, even though only two products come from elk farms: elk antler velvet, marketed as a miracle supplement and aphrodisiac, and "domestic trophies" for hunters who kill animals confined to pens. The elk antler velvet has an especially large market in Asia. And while most serious hunters frown upon elk farms, there are many who prefer to hunt an animal in a confined area. It is not much of a sport, but the fact remains that these farms have been successful.

Years ago, Beth Williams advised the Department of Agriculture in Colorado not to issue permits to new elk farms after the disease had been discovered in the area. She feared, rightly so, that it would facilitate the spread of the disease. Her pleas, as well as the pleas of other experts, were ignored. Now, taxpayers are funding a $15 million buyout of twenty Colorado elk ranches that most people said never should have been built in the first place.

The Future of Elk Farms

Unfortunately, the Colorado government has said nothing about banning elk ranches in the future. Critics of elk ranches suggest that these beautiful animals were meant to be out in the wild, and now, trying to domesticate and market them as a product has led to numerous problems. Elk are not just being slaughtered in captivity when one in a herd tests positive for CWD. There are also unfortunate animals in the wild that will get the disease through contact with sick elk through the fencing.

CWD has caused the destruction of thirty-eight elk ranches in the United States since 1997. Although elk ranching is a young industry, elk ranches have already been destroyed in six states—Colorado, Nebraska, Montana, Oklahoma, South Dakota, and Kansas—after an animal tested positive. More than 3,800 elk have been slaughtered in the United States on elk farms.

The United States Spreads CWD to Its Neighbor

CWD was first diagnosed in Canada in a farmed elk in 1996, most likely the result of an elk being imported from the United States. In 2000, Canada instituted a national program to deal with CWD. Any deer or elk showing signs of the disease is put to sleep and tested. If an animal at a game farm or ranch is identified with CWD, then all animals that have been exposed to it are

destroyed. Animals that have been exposed to an infected animal (before it is diagnosed) within the previous thirty-six to sixty months are kept under surveillance by vets until sixty months after the animal's last exposure. Because the infected animal can be symptom free for years, the strict precautions are viewed as necessary. In 2000 and 2001, 7,500 elk were destroyed in Canada. Of the 6,481 that were tested, 224 tested positive for CWD, but only 22 showed outward signs of the disease, according to the

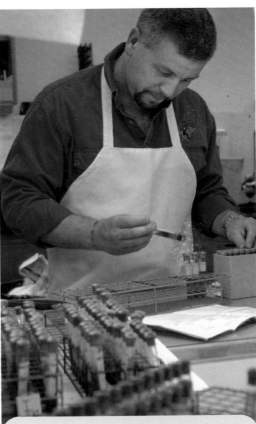

Technician Keith Bloss checks animal blood samples for CWD at the Wisconsin Veterinary Diagnostics Laboratory.

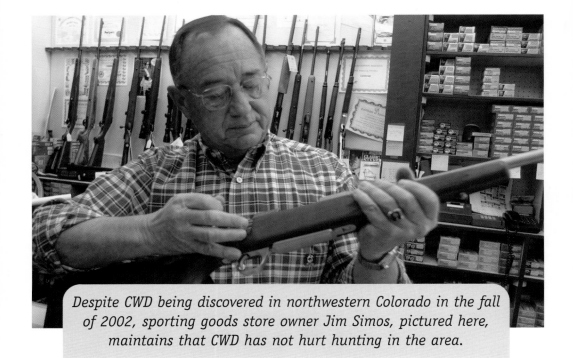

Despite CWD being discovered in northwestern Colorado in the fall of 2002, sporting goods store owner Jim Simos, pictured here, maintains that CWD has not hurt hunting in the area.

Canadian Food Inspection Agency in 2002. Since only 10 percent of animals that tested positive showed outward signs of CWD, you can see why experts fear that many infected animals are thought to be healthy. Since there is no accurate live test, many infected animals are viewed as healthy based only on visual clues.

Precautions Hunters Should Take

Government officials have spent the past few years informing hunters that they have nothing to fear from CWD. Hunting greatly contributes to the economy in many of the states where CWD has been discovered. Governments rely on hunters and the money they bring in. However, the risk that CWD poses is not being completely ignored. States have enacted numerous regulations for hunters and butchers. In addition, lobbyists are busy in the state capitals and in Washington, D.C., trying to secure money for more research on CWD. Currently, the state of Colorado has the most restrictions related to CWD. This is because Colorado has the highest infection rate of CWD in the wild and domestic populations of deer and elk. Although the disease is less prevalent in elk than deer, precautions communicated to the public and to hunters are the same. Hunters are advised to not shoot, handle, or consume any animal that appears to be sick. When dealing with a carcass, people are instructed to wear rubber gloves and have minimal contact with the animal's brain or spinal cord. After field dressing, or handling the carcass once the animal has been killed, hunters are told to thoroughly wash their hands and instruments, preferably with bleach.

Testing and Government Restrictions

Most states where CWD has been identified have set up some type of testing program. Participation by hunters is mandatory in some areas and voluntary in others. In areas where CWD is not monitored, hunters may choose to send the head of their kill to the Colorado State University laboratory or the Wyoming state veterinary laboratory where it will be tested. These labs will send results to the hunter, usually within six to eight weeks.

Researchers and biologists are desperately seeking more information about CWD. In the meantime, local officials are trying to prevent the spread of CWD beyond areas where it has already been identified, as well as trying to eradicate the disease within those areas. Officials are attempting to reduce the number of deer and elk in diseased herds by hiring sharpshooters to slaughter them. Since the transport of animals within or between states has often spread CWD, governments are also attempting to strictly enforce the transport laws from game farms and to limit movement of herds between states.

Sharpshooters Try to Eliminate Herds

The most controversial policy instituted has been the hiring of sharpshooters to kill deer in areas where the infection rate is very high. Hunters have been upset

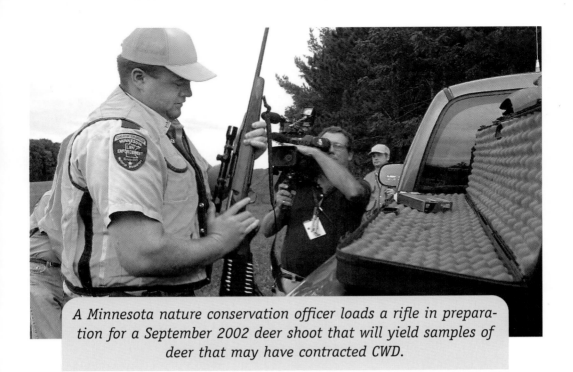

A Minnesota nature conservation officer loads a rifle in preparation for a September 2002 deer shoot that will yield samples of deer that may have contracted CWD.

because the sharpshooters sometimes arrive right before hunting season. Deer killed by government sharpshooters are dumped in a landfill where they are left to rot, which also upsets people. In addition to the problem of the smell of rotting carcasses, nobody has yet been able to guarantee that the dead animals don't pose a health risk. There is speculation that CWD could evolve into variants, like mad cow disease did. Landfills are often populated by flocks of birds—vultures, hawks, crows, and seagulls. Some may land on the animal pile. Who knows what they are eating? Who knows how it is affecting them? Unfortunately, no facility in areas of high infection would have the

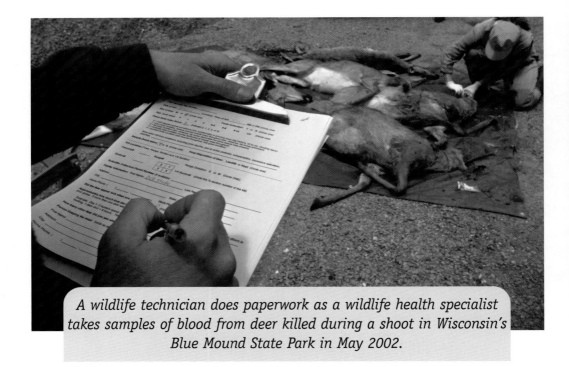

A wildlife technician does paperwork as a wildlife health specialist takes samples of blood from deer killed during a shoot in Wisconsin's Blue Mound State Park in May 2002.

capacity to incinerate the animals either. There are no easy solutions available.

Live Tests

Since no live test (a test on a live animal) for CWD is currently available, drastic measures taken to curb the spread of the disease have come under heavy criticism. Since sick animals can appear healthy, it cannot be determined easily which herds are infected. Large numbers of healthy deer and elk have been killed for testing, in the hopes of preventing the spread of CWD. Fortunately, experts are optimistic that a live test will soon be available. This one advancement could help the needless slaughter of animals on game farms and in limited situations in the wild. However, even with a live test, it may take weeks to calculate the results. While this would greatly help game farms and domestic herds, it is impractical to think that entire wild herds could be detained while the tests are processed in a laboratory hundreds of miles away.

3

SCIENCE

Despite all the recent attention being given to chronic wasting disease, there are still many more questions about the disease than answers. What we do know is that CWD is a neurological disease that affects both wild and captive deer and elk. We also know that CWD is always fatal.

Symptoms of CWD

Once a deer or elk contracts CWD, the animal can remain symptom free for a number of years. Studies report that the time between an animal contracting the disease and developing visible symptoms is one to five years. After symptoms do begin to occur, the animal will not live for long. Progressive weight loss follows, and the animal starts to behave strangely, including constantly grinding its teeth. The animal drinks very large amounts of water and urinates and salivates excessively. Animals in captivity with CWD have been studied and have shown repetitive movements, an avoidance of other animals, lowering of the head, and apparent stupor.

In the wild, animals that normally fear humans do not. Strangely, infected animals also begin to fear things that they normally don't fear, such as other animals. CWD-infected deer and elk often shake and are very weak. There is no cure or treatment for CWD. If an animal gets infected, it will die. The only question is how long it may live with the disease before the onset of symptoms. Once symptoms begin, the animal's days are numbered.

Transmission

Scientists are baffled as to how the disease is transmitted. They just aren't sure. They think it is most likely transmitted through direct contact between animals. Along with direct contact, scientists also think that CWD can be transmitted through contamination of feed or water sources with saliva, urine, or feces. It seems the disease occurs most frequently in places where animals are crowded or where they gather at man-made feed or water stations, something often seen on game farms and elk ranches.

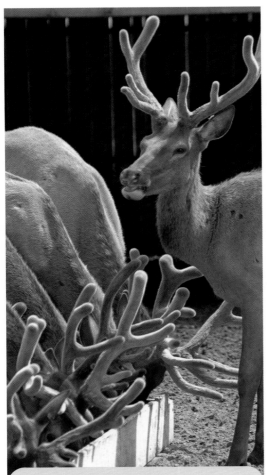

Elk raised for their antler velvet drink at a watering station, which can be a breeding ground for CWD.

Diagnosis

A definite diagnosis of CWD can be made only after an animal's death. The brain must be examined to determine if it has undergone the typical spongiform changes associated with CWD that result in a spongelike appearance. A current live test of an animal's tonsils has been proven effective in deer but unfortunately not in elk. Now, experts must figure out how to use the test in the field on wild animals.

Under ideal laboratory conditions, once a test has begun, it takes slightly longer than two days to determine if a deer or elk is infected.

Because of CWD's long incubation period, the infected brain can sometimes look healthy under a microscope. The postmortem brain examination is still the most widely done test, so even animals that test negative could actually be positive and in the very early stages of the disease. A more sensitive chemical test is being developed that researchers believe could detect the disease within six months of infection. Yet another experimental test shows promise of detecting the disease forty-two days after infection, but approval of these tests is a long way off.

CWD Is Caused by Prions

CWD is not a virus or bacteria like most other diseases. Most experts believe that CWD is caused by something called a prion. There are two types of proteins in the brains of diseased animals. One is a normal protein found in all mammals. The other is a disease-causing form, called a prion. It is chemically identical to the original protein, but has a different shape, which makes it resistant to heat and disinfectants. It has no genetic material. Once in its abnormal form, the prion can corrupt healthy proteins it comes into contact with, turning them into prions. So, the prions are not replicating themselves; they are converting healthy proteins, which causes an infected animal to become sick. When enough infected prions deposit themselves in the brain, microscopic ruptures form in brain cells that affect behavior, as with all TSEs. Experts are having trouble finding a cure for CWD and TSEs in general because there is nothing to kill. There is no genetic material to destroy.

Even though it is widely recognized that prions are the cause of CWD, there are two other possible theories that a few scientists have suggested. Some researchers feel CWD may be an unconventional virus that is resistant to treatment and also does not behave like conventional viruses. The other theory proposes that CWD may be an "incomplete" virus composed of nucleic acid protected by host proteins. Since the CWD agent would be smaller than most viral particles, it would not create an immune response in the host, as would be expected.

Why TSEs Are Such a Problem

Bacteria or viruses are tiny microbes that cause most diseases and can only be seen under a microscope. Bacteria and viruses contain genetic material—nucleic acid, like DNA. DNA is the basic template for protein production. Nucleic acid is the necessary ingredient of life and allows organisms to reproduce. Bacteria and viruses cause disease by spreading toxins or damaging their host.

TSEs are different from any other disease and therefore have confused scientists since their discovery. They cause no immune response in the body. Since no antibodies are produced, there is no sign that the body is fighting an infection. TSEs defy the rules of biology. Radiation, which kills viruses and bacteria by destroying their genetic material, has no effect on TSEs since they have no genetic material. Since TSEs follow no laws of biology, scientists do not know how to fight them. Scientists can neither stop nor slow the effects of a TSE.

Prions Are Almost Impossible to Destroy

In areas where CWD has been confirmed, prions have contaminated the ground and remain contractible by other animals for many years. In one pen, where captive animals were held and contracted CWD, all the animals were slaughtered. The ground was plowed, then sprayed with bleach that experts thought was strong enough to kill the prions. One year later, twelve calves were placed in the pens. Within five years, two had died of CWD.

Researchers have found that TSE prions are nearly indestructible. Prions cannot be destroyed through cooking or normal sterilization. When doctors perform

Stanley Prusiner, a San Francisco neurologist and micro-biologist, has done most of the research on prions and TSEs. Prusiner developed his theory on prions by conducting experiments so different from conventional science that other scientists thought he was crazy. In 1997, Prusiner received the Nobel Prize in medicine. Few question his theories anymore. His research has given scientists most of the little information that they have on prions and TSEs.

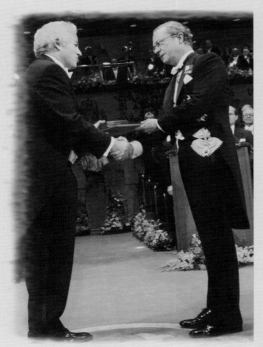

King Carl XVI Gustaf (right) *of Sweden presents Stanley B. Prusiner with the Nobel Prize for medicine at the Concert Hall in Stockholm, Sweden. Prusiner's work on TSEs and prions has been groundbreaking.*

autopsies on people who died of Creutzfeldt-Jakob disease (a TSE that naturally affects humans), they wear two sets of gloves, gowns, masks, and eye shields and take every other possible precaution. Hospitals use stronger disinfectants and higher temperatures to sterilize their equipment as well. The temperature needed to kill prions is 680° Fahrenheit (360° Celsius). In one test, prions caused infection in test animals after surviving for three years in an empty concrete cell where diseased animals were once held.

The origin and life cycle of prions are the target of ongoing research. Since most scientists believe that prions are responsible for CWD and other TSEs, learning more about them is essential. Ultimately, by learning about prions, scientists hope to develop a plan to eliminate and contain the prions in captive herds and in the wild.

4

WHY IS IT AN EPIDEMIC?

With confirmed cases numbering only in the hundreds, why is CWD considered an epidemic? CWD is spreading rapidly, and as it continues to spread, many more animals are at risk for exposure. It is now being discovered where most people thought it wasn't possible—west of the Rockies and east of the Mississippi. CWD prions are extremely difficult to kill and very hard to identify. What is most frightening is that we are not sure if the disease can be transmitted to humans in the future as CWD or a variant disease, like CJD. Most scientists agree that it is a long shot that humans can be affected by CWD, but no one will go so far as to say it's impossible.

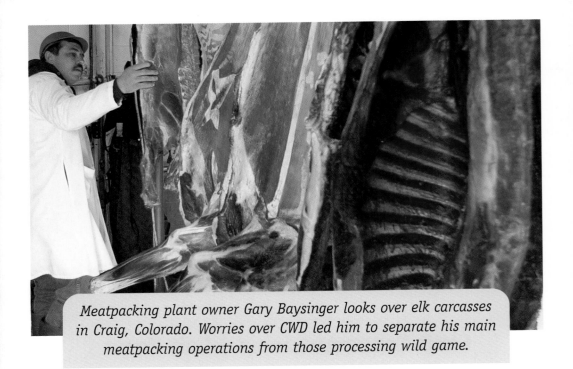

Meatpacking plant owner Gary Baysinger looks over elk carcasses in Craig, Colorado. Worries over CWD led him to separate his main meatpacking operations from those processing wild game.

All TSEs Are Fatal

Experts have the most fear about things they don't know or can't explain. With CWD and all TSEs, what is not known about the diseases far outweighs what is known. Currently, all diseases classified as TSEs have no known cure. If you get the disease, you will die.

At first CWD was viewed more as a curiosity, something that occurred in some deer and elk in small numbers. It was also concentrated in just two states—Colorado and Wyoming—for almost thirty years. Then came the rapid spread of cases of vCJD in the United States and the mad cow epidemic in England. Once a

TSE made the leap from cows to humans, experts became very concerned. A disease thought to be found only in cows had made the "species jump." Humans who had eaten meat or meat products from cows with BSE were getting sick and dying. CWD and BSE were both TSEs, so was it crazy to think the unthinkable? Can CWD make the species jump into cows and threaten America's huge cattle ranches, or worse, could it affect humans who eat deer or elk infected with CWD? The results could be catastrophic.

CWD Transmission in Lab Tests

Although immediate tests have shown that CWD could not affect humans, some experts aren't so sure. In laboratory conditions, human cells can be infected by CWD through a process in which CWD is directly injected into human cells. There is, however, no proof that this can occur naturally. As for CWD affecting cattle, tests are ongoing. When kept in close proximity to deer with CWD, no cattle have been infected. When CWD prions were injected directly into the brains of thirteen test cows, three became infected. So, as with humans, there is some cause for concern. While it is frightening that CWD has been transmitted to other species during lab tests, no test has shown that infection can occur any other way. Studies are being made

In 1996, it was confirmed that mad cow disease migrated to humans and affected them as vCJD. From that point on, the Centers for Disease Control and Prevention (CDC) began searching for an increase in TSE-like diseases in humans in the United States. Specifically, the CDC searched for variations of CJD, which is what mad cow disease became when it made the species jump. Only one case of CJD in 270 million occurs annually in people under age thirty in the United States. The average age of CJD victims is sixty-eight. Any case in which a young person got the disease was investigated. In the last few years, the CDC has investigated all cases of young people who contracted CJD, including cases among some hunters, but no link to CWD has been confirmed. But the tests being done may not be conclusive. As one expert, Michael Hansen, a Consumers Union scientist, explained in a 2002 *Rocky Mountain News* article, "If CWD infected a human brain, we wouldn't know what it would look like."

in which infected animals are in close contact with cattle and other animals, and to date, there has been no natural mode of transmission between species.

Incorrect Information

Everyone agrees that the government response to mad cow disease was flawed in England. The British government insisted for years that there was no threat to humans. The government claimed people could eat diseased beef and beef products and wouldn't get sick. The government was wrong.

Similarly, there have been problems with the United States government keeping people informed about CWD. There are also people convinced that officials are dragging their feet and giving incomplete or incorrect information to the public. The deer and elk industry in the Midwest is a multimillion-dollar industry. Hunters come in during hunting season and fuel a huge tourist industry. There are too many people with an interest in maintaining the tourist and hunter dollars coming into their state. If there is panic among hunters and butchers, an industry could be greatly affected in that region.

Currently, there are numerous restrictions being placed on hunters. Officials in states where CWD has been found also give warnings to hunters on a regular basis. In 1998, as a precaution, state officials in Colorado (where the disease is found most often) started to caution hunters about eating brain and spinal cord material from deer and elk. Experts feel that prions are most likely to accumulate in the eyes, tonsils, lymph nodes, spleen, brain, and spinal cord. Two years of government statements followed in which officials insisted there was no danger to humans and no need for concern, that CWD wasn't spreading. In reality, it was spreading faster than anyone had anticipated.

For years, it was difficult to convince people that CWD was something very serious that they should fear. Until recently, many states only monitored the growth of CWD but did little else to pre-vent its spread or to erad-icate it. Thus far, the government response to CWD in the United States has been similar to the British response to mad cow disease years ago. The wrong information in England that was provided to the public caused the deaths of many people.

Are Hunters Most at Risk?

We often talk about the danger to hunters who consume the meat of infected animals. In 2001, in the two states

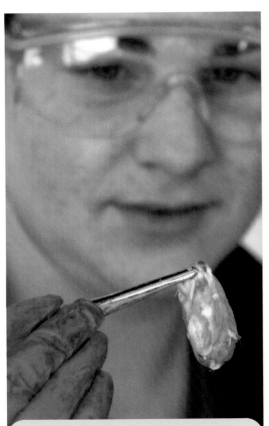

A Colorado wildlife technician holds up an elk's lymph node, which will be tested for CWD.

where CWD is most prevalent, hunters killed many animals. In Colorado, only in the endemic area, hunters killed more than 2,100 deer and 1,262 elk. In endemic southern Wyoming, hunters killed 5,497 deer and 798 elk, according to a *Rocky Mountain News* article in 2002. In all likelihood, the hunters consumed hundreds of thousands of pounds of the meat, and shared it with family and friends.

Hunters have been consuming infected deer for a while, and there has been no known link between eating infected meat and a resulting disease in humans. But if only a few of the thousands of hunters that consumed the meat got infected, as happened in England with beef, it may take years for scientists to notice.

Scientists Baffled by TSEs

Another possibility being explored is of CWD infecting another species, changing characteristics, and then infecting humans. It's not likely, but it's certainly possible. While we still have so many questions about the disease, all possibilities are frightening and must be researched. But research costs money, and right now scientists need more of it.

The more scientists find out about TSEs, the more concerned they are. As mentioned earlier, TSEs

Dr. Thomas Pringle, a molecular biologist who for five years worked on TSE research in Oregon, has serious doubts about government claims. Dr. Pringle argues that for years game agencies in Colorado and Wyoming have assured people that there is no proof anyone ever died from eating CWD-tainted venison, yet there is no research to back up their claims. He believes that the research on potential human health risks is nonexistent and that their position has been taken to protect a multimillion-dollar industry that revolves around deer and elk hunting.

don't follow any laws of science. A recent paper documented a study done on rodents. Researchers took brains of hamsters infected with scrapie prions and injected the brain tissue into the neural tissue of the lab mice. The mice were killed at various intervals and all tested negative for the replication of the mutant prions. From the supposedly prion-free mice, researchers took brain matter and injected it into another set of healthy mice and hamsters. These rodents soon developed TSEs and died. So the first set, despite testing negative, weren't free of prions after all.

The fact that carriers can test negative and appear symptom free is very scary. It could mean

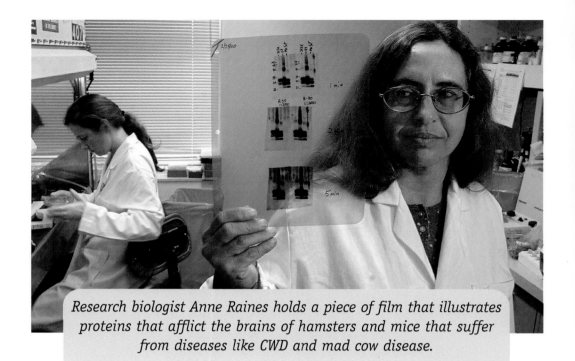

Research biologist Anne Raines holds a piece of film that illustrates proteins that afflict the brains of hamsters and mice that suffer from diseases like CWD and mad cow disease.

that the number of people in Europe infected with mad cow disease could be far greater than anyone anticipates. Maybe many people are currently infected without showing signs. There could be huge amounts of people who are currently carriers of vCJD without having any symptoms whatsoever. Could they unknowingly be spreading the disease? The possibilities are staggering. There could be thousands of people with low levels of prions converting healthy proteins into harmful ones. Again, we just don't know.

Most scientists will say that it is unlikely that CWD can be transmitted to humans. Just a few years ago, before mad cow disease began to kill humans in the form of vCJD, those same scientists would have laughed at the notion that CWD could harm us. Clearly, today everyone is proceeding with a lot more caution after what happened in England. It is not until more research is done that we will be able to say for sure what the effects of the disease will be.

5

WHAT THE FUTURE HOLDS

The future of chronic wasting disease is uncertain. It will most certainly continue to spread geographically until considerably more research is done. Most likely you will be hearing about it on the news more than you ever did before. This will make a greater amount of people aware of the disease. Because of this, hopefully, government officials will give funds for additional research and education. More work must be done. Thus far, aside from a few states whose economies are being affected, progress has been very slow.

CWD and the Midwest Economy

The economic impact of CWD will be far reaching if the spread of the disease continues

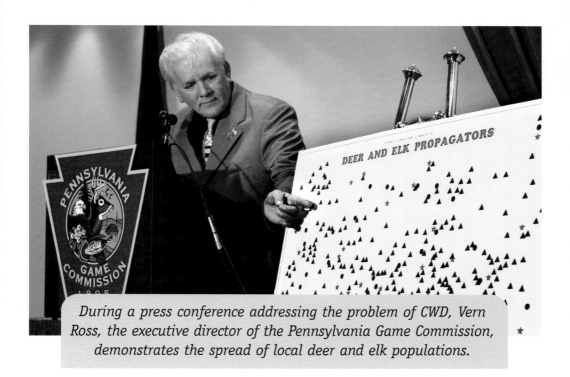

During a press conference addressing the problem of CWD, Vern Ross, the executive director of the Pennsylvania Game Commission, demonstrates the spread of local deer and elk populations.

unchecked. States such as Colorado and Wyoming are known for their abundant wildlife and gain their identity from it. Animals will be lost due to the depopulation of herds, and governments will have to spend a great deal of money on surveillance programs. Tourist revenue will be affected in certain areas, and markets for meat and antler velvet will be hurt. There are more than 500,000 deer and 250,000 elk in Colorado. It is a premier area for hunters and watchers of wildlife. It is estimated that hunters are responsible for contributing $600 million to local economies each year. This includes the purchase of equipment, lodging, gasoline, and other things related to their hunt. The Colorado Division of Wildlife is also dependent on the sale of hunting licenses for its annual $85 million budget. If there are no hunters, where will the money come from?

What Is Colorado Doing?

In Colorado, the state's chief goals have been to minimize any panic and yet preserve the hunting industry. This must be done while reporting everything it knows about the disease without fear of how the public will respond. Leaving the responsibility of public awareness to the Division of Wildlife may have contributed to the spread—not because of any malicious motive, but because of the agency's function and tradition. The division exists to manage wildlife and is funded by the purchase of hunting and fishing licenses. Somehow, a way must be found to pass honest information to the public without conflict-of-interest issues. The Division of Wildlife also hopes to stop the spread of CWD beyond historically infected areas. Some herds need to be eradicated and other herds need to have diseased animals removed. Illegal feeding regulations and transport laws must be enforced to restrict movement of deer and elk from infected areas.

Research Is Critical

Research is needed not only for CWD but also for all TSEs. There are links between the diseases, where research being done on one disease could prove vital to gaining answers about another. Further study could also save human lives. Research on prions and misshapen proteins could give scientists answers to more widespread diseases like Alzheimer's and Parkinson's and could lead to new treatments. Unfortunately, emphasis is being placed on each disease as a separate entity, not on linking similarities between them. This must change.

During the next few years, research will be the most important thing we can do. A live test is desperately needed, as are improved and more sensitive tests on animals that have died. Studies must be done to determine if the disease spreads more rapidly in deer herds that populate a small area. More research on diagnosis of CWD and transmission is also needed. We need to know if it can be spread to sheep, mountain lions, cattle, and other animals. Most important, we need to know if there is a link between the consumption of infected meat and the development of neurological disease in humans. The studies that must be done to determine if humans can be

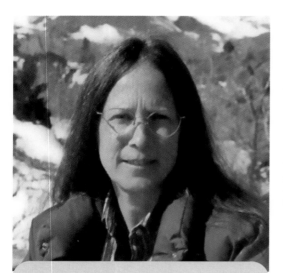

Veterinarian Beth Williams, pictured here, is considered one of the leading authorities on CWD research.

affected by CWD also raise issues with animal rights activists. Controversial research using primates may be needed. Such studies are costly and distasteful to many people, but they could be very helpful.

Testing Needs to Be Improved

The live animal test is one of the keys for the future. The only current live test involves removing part of the animal's tonsil. Unfortunately, this is time consuming and impractical when dealing with hundreds of animals. A live test will be most important in dealing with farms. It would prevent the needless slaughter of hundreds of animals that reside on farms, where only one may be confirmed as CWD positive.

Today, hunters wait up to eight weeks to learn whether their kill had CWD after they send in a head for testing. Laboratory testing must be improved. It is not fair for hunters to wait this long for test

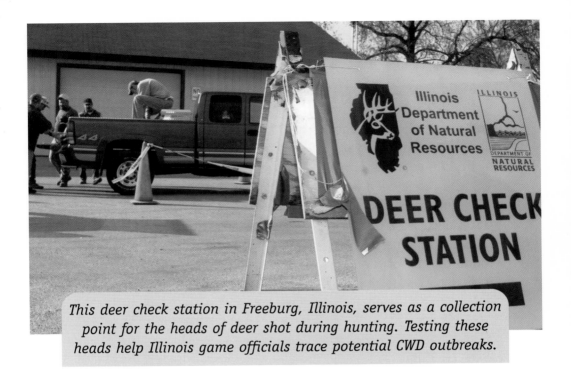

This deer check station in Freeburg, Illinois, serves as a collection point for the heads of deer shot during hunting. Testing these heads help Illinois game officials trace potential CWD outbreaks.

results. It has been suggested that mobile testing stations in popular hunting areas could be used during hunting season. The mobile stations would enable hunters to get quick results of the health of their animals before eating the meat, provided a rapid test is discovered and approved.

Government Officials Need to Be Informed

Right now, experts are not sure about much when dealing with CWD. They need to be sure. Saying that "there is nothing to show that CWD can be

The United States Department of Agriculture (USDA) is the national agency that has the most involvement with CWD and the public. This agency has been doing testing and has been working with various local governments in the hopes of finding common ground in the eradication of the disease. The USDA has been active in working with states with CWD programs and will continue to do so. In September 2001, the USDA declared a CWD emergency nationwide and announced its plans to wipe out the disease. Even though CWD was not found on any of the game farms in the Colorado area where it is most widespread, the USDA bought the farms and destroyed all the elk as a preventive measure.

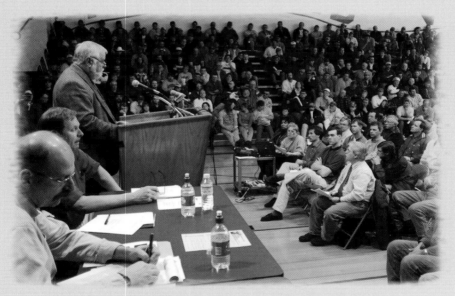

A crowd of 1,000 gathered in Mt. Horeb, Wisconsin, on March 20, 2002, to discuss CWD outbreaks in the state's deer population. Local agencies worked closely with federal agencies like the USDA to stem the tide of CWD.

transmitted to humans" is very different than saying "it can't be transmitted." If scientists say that there's no evidence that humans can get sick from eating meat from deer that are infected, why are they telling us not to eat certain parts of that deer? Research cannot be stopped until all of these questions are answered. To do this will take millions of dollars. Officials must be made aware of the danger of CWD even in areas where CWD has not yet been identified. They must know the disease is spreading rapidly. They must be told that it is not known how CWD spreads, that there is no cure, and that humans may very well be at risk.

If we all stay informed and the proper funding is made available, hopefully these questions will all be answered in a few years. Otherwise, we have every right to fear chronic wasting disease since so little is known and it may do so much damage in the future.

GLOSSARY

agent Something that produces or is capable of producing an effect.

aphrodisiac Something that arouses or is believed to arouse sexual desire.

barrier Something that blocks or is intended to block passage.

captivity State of being captive or kept within bounds.

convert To alter the physical or chemical nature of something; to change from one form or function to another.

domesticate To adapt an animal to life in close association with humans.

endemic Restricted or peculiar to a locality or region.

host A living animal or plant that allows a parasite or pathogen to live off of it.

incinerate To burn to ashes.

inflammation An irregular condition of some part of the body resulting from injury or infection, characterized by pain, heat, redness, and/or swelling.

mandatory Required.

neurological Pertaining to the nervous system, including the brain or spinal cord.

plausible Seemingly true or worthy of belief.

precaution A measure taken beforehand to prevent harm; safeguard.

prevalent Widespread.

primate The group of mammals including apes, monkeys, and related forms.

replicate To produce a copy.

sterilization The act of cleansing an object or area of harmful organisms.

supplement Something that completes or makes an addition.

variant Different in some way from others of the same type or class.

voluntary Proceeding from one's own choice or consent.

FOR MORE INFORMATION

In the United States

Colorado Division of Wildlife
6060 Broadway
Denver, CO 80216
(303) 297-1192
Web site: http://wildlife.state.co.us

Colorado Wildlife Federation
P.O. Box 280967
Lakewood, CO 80228
(303) 987-0400
Web site: http://www.coloradowildlife.org

Mule Deer Foundation
1005 Terminal Way, Suite 170
Reno, NV 89502

(775) 322-6558
Web site: http://www.muledeer.org

Rocky Mountain Elk Foundation
P.O. Box 8249
Missoula, MT 59807-8249
(406) 523-4543
Web site: http://www.rmef.org

Quality Deer Management Association
P.O. Box 227
Watkinsville, GA 30677
(800) 209-3337
Web site: http://www.qdma.org

Wildlife Management Institute
1101 14th Street NW, Suite 801
Washington, DC 20005
(202) 371-1808
Web site: http://www.wildlifemanagementinstitute.org

In Canada

Canadian Food Inspection Agency
59 Camelot Drive
Ottawa, ON K1A 0Y9
(613) 225-2342
(800) 442-2342
Web site: http://www.inspection.gc.ca

Web Sites

Due to the changing nature of Internet links, the Rosen Publishing Group, Inc., has developed an online list of Web sites related to the subject of this book. This site is updated regularly. Please use this link to access the list:

http://www.rosenlinks.com/epid/chwd

FOR FURTHER READING

Berger, Todd R., ed. *Majestic Elk: The Ultimate Tribute to North America's Greatest Game Animal.* Stillwater, MN: Voyageur Press, 2001.

Richey, David. *The Ultimate Guide to Deer Hunting.* New York: Lyons Press, 2001.

Robinson, Jerome B. *In the Deer Woods: Tips, Tactics and Adventure Tales of Hunting for Whitetails, Mulies, Moose, Elk and Caribou.* New York: Lyons Press, 2000.

Roy, Jim. *Real World Whitetail Behavior.* Revised edition. Lanham, MD: Derrydale Press, 2003.

INDEX

B

bacteria, 34–35

bovine spongiform encephalopathy (BSE; mad cow disease), 10–11, 27, 40, 41

outbreak in England of, 11–12, 39, 41–42, 43, 44, 46, 47

brain, effects of TSEs on, 9–10, 34

C

Canada, CWD in, 17, 22–24

Canadian Food Inspection Agency, 24

Centers for Disease Control and Prevention, 41

Cheesebro, Bruce, 20–21

chronic wasting disease (CWD)

cause of, 33–34, 37

cure/treatment for, 31, 34, 39, 55

diagnosis of, 32–33

economic impact of, 48–50

and humans, 38, 40, 44, 46–47, 51–52, 53–55

symptoms of, 30–31

transmission of, 12, 18, 31–32

Colorado,

CWD in, 16, 17, 18, 25, 39

elk ranches in, 21, 22, 54

hunting in, 25, 42, 44, 45, 49, 50

Colorado Division of Wildlife, 5, 50

Creutzfeldt-Jakob disease (CJD), 11, 36, 38, 41

D

deer, CWD and, 8, 11, 12–13, 16, 17, 23, 25, 26, 30, 31, 32, 40, 51, 55

DNA, 34

CREDITS

About the Authors

Gregory Payan is a freelance author living in Forest Hills, New York. Casey Gallagher is an aspiring veterinary student whose stepfather is president of the South Carolina chapter of the Rocky Mountain Elk Foundation.

Photo Credits

Cover and chapter title interior photos and page 52 Beth Williams, University of Wyoming; pp. 4, 23, 54 © Andy Manis/AP/Wide World Photos; p. 11 © Alastair Grant/AP/Wide World Photos; p. 13 © Jack Dempsey/AP/Wide World Photos; p. 19 © *Akron Beacon Journal*/Bob Demay/AP/Wide World Photos; pp. 24, 39, 43 © Ed Anrieski/AP/Wide World Photos; p. 27 © *Duluth News Tribune*, Renee Knoeber/AP/Wide World Photos; p. 28 © *Wisconsin State Journal*, Steve Apps/AP/Wide World Photos; p. 32 © Joan Seidel/AP/Wide World Photos; p. 36 © Jonas Ekstromer/AP/Wide World Photos; p. 46 © Tom Bauer, *Missoulian*/AP/Wide World Photos; p. 49 © Paul Vathis/AP/Wide World Photos; p. 53 © *Belleville News-Democrat*/Derik Holtmann/AP/Wide World Photos.

Designer: Evelyn Horovicz; Editor: Eliza Berkowitz

12109

573.8
PAY   Payan, Gregory

         Chronic wasting
         disease

573.8
PAY   Payan, Gregory

         Chronic wasting
         disease

BRODART   10/04   26.50

12109